Nathália Sorrini Fujita
Patrícia da Graça Leite Speridião

ANCTEA

Nathália Sorrini Fujita
Patrícia da Graça Leite Speridião

ANCTEA

NUTRITIONAL CARE FOR CHILDREN WITH AUTISM SPECTRUM DISORDER

ScienciaScripts

Imprint

Any brand names and product names mentioned in this book are subject to trademark, brand or patent protection and are trademarks or registered trademarks of their respective holders. The use of brand names, product names, common names, trade names, product descriptions etc. even without a particular marking in this work is in no way to be construed to mean that such names may be regarded as unrestricted in respect of trademark and brand protection legislation and could thus be used by anyone.

Cover image: www.ingimage.com

This book is a translation from the original published under ISBN 978-620-6-75827-3.

Publisher:
Sciencia Scripts
is a trademark of
Dodo Books Indian Ocean Ltd. and OmniScriptum S.R.L publishing group

120 High Road, East Finchley, London, N2 9ED, United Kingdom
Str. Armeneasca 28/1, office 1, Chisinau MD-2012, Republic of Moldova, Europe
Printed at: see last page
ISBN: 978-620-7-63470-5

AUTHORS

Nahália Sorrini Fujita

Nutritionist, graduated from Universidade Estadual Paulista (UNESP) - Instituto de Biociências - Botucatu. Specialist in Child Health from the Pontifical Catholic University (PUC) - Campinas. Specialist in Clinical Neurology in Rehabilitation at the Federal University of São Paulo (UNIFESP) – São Paulo. Postgraduate course in progress at the Professional Master's Degree in Teaching in Health Sciences at the Escola Paulista de Enfermagem of the Federal University of São Paulo (UNIFESP). Nutritionist at the Specialized Rehabilitation Centre (CER) in the municipality of Barueri.

Patrícia da Graça Leite Speridião Nutritionist. Professor. Professor in the Nutrition Course at the Federal University of São Paulo - Health and Society Institute and in the Postgraduate Program in Professional Master's in Teaching in Health Sciences at the Paulista School of Nursing at the Federal University of São Paulo.

PRESENTATION

The purpose of this *e-book is* to go beyond providing information on the aspects that permeate nutritional care for children with Autism Spectrum Disorder (ASD).

This *e-book* is based on the scarcity of similar material, as well as the limited knowledge and practice of health professionals at a Specialized Rehabilitation Center (CER).

Thus, this *e-book* was designed to help health professionals understand the need for nutritional assistance for children with ASD, both in terms of knowledge and clinical practice.

It is hoped that this material will fill this gap in the knowledge and practice of nutritional care for children with ASD and may provoke other researchers to look into the subject.

The authors.

CHAPTER 1.

Nutritional Care

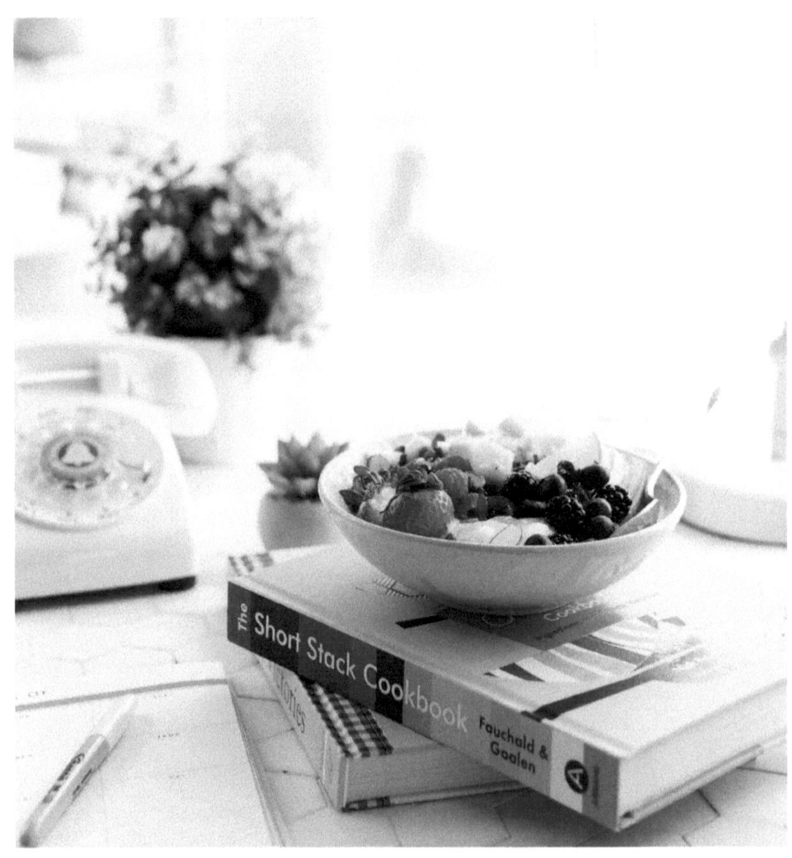

The field of nutrition in Brazil came to the fore in the 1930s, during a period of world war in which the population had great difficulty in obtaining food. Many began to live in unfavorable situations, such as hunger and poverty, which had a negative impact on their health and survival.

Faced with this scenario, it was necessary to promote the training of health professionals who could help continuously and effectively, not only with prevention and the most frequent health care at the time, until the profession of Nutritionist emerged. The nutritionist is the professional qualified to plan and guide individuals in all areas related to food and nutrition, both in the health-disease care process and in promotion, prevention and recovery actions, in order to provide healthier living and eating habits.

Nutritional Care (NC) is defined as all the care involved in food and nutrition, from health promotion actions to the treatment of illnesses, and the protagonists of NC should be patients, their families and the community, based on the construction of a network of integrality and humanization of care.

In this context, it is worth highlighting the existence of multiple scenarios experienced by the Brazilian population, including discrepancies between obesity and malnutrition, the prevalence of chronic non-communicable diseases (CNCDs), as well as the vulnerable situation of many families due to the lack of subsidies for food and nutritional security, considering age groups and specific health conditions. These conditions make it increasingly necessary for actions to be articulated between all spheres of government and the comprehensive health care network, whether in Primary Care (PC), secondary care (outpatient clinics) or tertiary care (hospitals).

Adequate nutrition and the right to quality food are elementary and basic rights, according to the Federal Constitution and the Universal Declaration of Human Rights. Food and nutrition are part of the requirements for health promotion and protection.

The AN is part of the National Food and Nutrition Policy (PNAN), as the first guiding guideline in the process of organization and implementation, initially in the Health Care Networks (RAS).

Among the public policies of great relevance to this context in the country, the PNAN is the one that proposes actions to promote, protect, prevent and treat health-disease issues, such as NCDs.

The actions proposed by the PNAN to tackle nutritional problems in the different contexts of the Brazilian population include those of greater interventionist complexity. This public policy was approved in 1999 by the Ministry of Health with the aim of combating hunger, poverty and food shortages. However, currently, in the nutritional transition, there is a change in the epidemiological profile, contrasting malnutrition and nutritional deficiencies with the alarming numbers of overweight and obesity and CNCDs. With this change in the nutritional transition, a new nutritional challenge arises in the context of this affected population.

There are 7 guidelines that make up the PNAN:
1) stimulating intersectoral actions for universal access to food; 2) guaranteeing food safety and quality; 3) monitoring the population's food and nutrition situation; 4) promoting healthy practices in the food sector; 5) preventing and controlling nutritional alterations and diseases associated with food and nutrition; 6) promoting the development of lines of research and; 7) developing and training human resources.

Faced with society's nutritional challenges, it is important to emphasize that the use of strategies aimed at protecting health based on care related to food and nutrition, including diagnosis, treatment of nutritional problems and prevention, associated with the health care actions of the Unified Health System (SUS), such as AN.

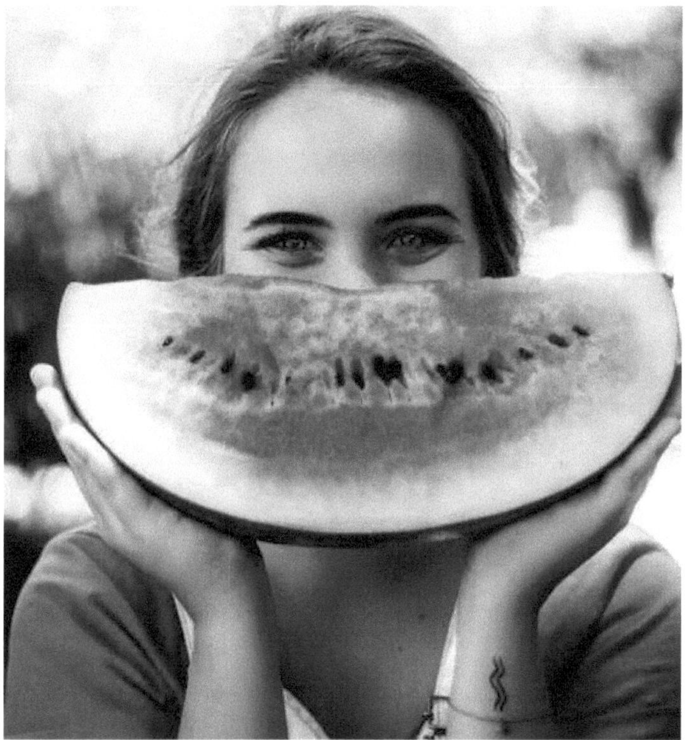

Among the actions of nutritional care, it is possible to carry out emancipatory education, with emphasis on Food and Nutrition Education (FNE). EAN is established as a tool for promoting health, healthy eating and changing eating habits, since it is an intersectoral, transdisciplinary and multiprofessional field, permeated by different approaches and perceptions, enabling the implementation of educational actions that contribute significantly to a better prognosis.

REFERENCES

BRAZIL. CFN RESOLUTION NO. 689, OF MAY 4, 2010

2021. Regulates the recognition of specialties in Nutrition and the registration, within the scope of the CFN/CRN System, of specialist titles for nutritionists. May/21.

FERRAZ LF. Nutrition in Brazil: emergence, regulation and forms of organization, mobilization and struggle of workers, in the city of Rio de Janeiro. 2019. Dissertation (Professional Master's Degree in Professional Health Education). Joaquim Venâncio Polytechnic Health School, Oswaldo Cruz Foundation. Rio de Janeiro. 2019.

FRANÇA CJ, SANTOS VCH. Food and nutrition education strategies in Primary Health Care: a literature review. Saúde em Debate. 2017; 114(41).

MINISTRY OF HEALTH AND SOCIAL SECURITY. Plan National Food and Nutrition Program PNAN 2021-2025. 2020.

PRADO BG, FORTES ENS, LOPES MAL. Actions of food and nutrition education for schoolchildren: an experience report. Demetra. 2016;11(2):369-382.

SOUZA LMS, SANTOS SMC. National Food and Nutrition Policy: evaluation of the implementation of programs in municipalities in Bahia. Demetra: alimentação, nutrição & saúde. 2017; 12(1); 137-155.

VASCONCELOS FAG, CALADO CLA. Profession nutritionist: 70 years of history in Brazil. Revista de Nutrição. 2011; 24(4): 605-617.

CHAPTER 2.

Autistic Spectrum Disorder

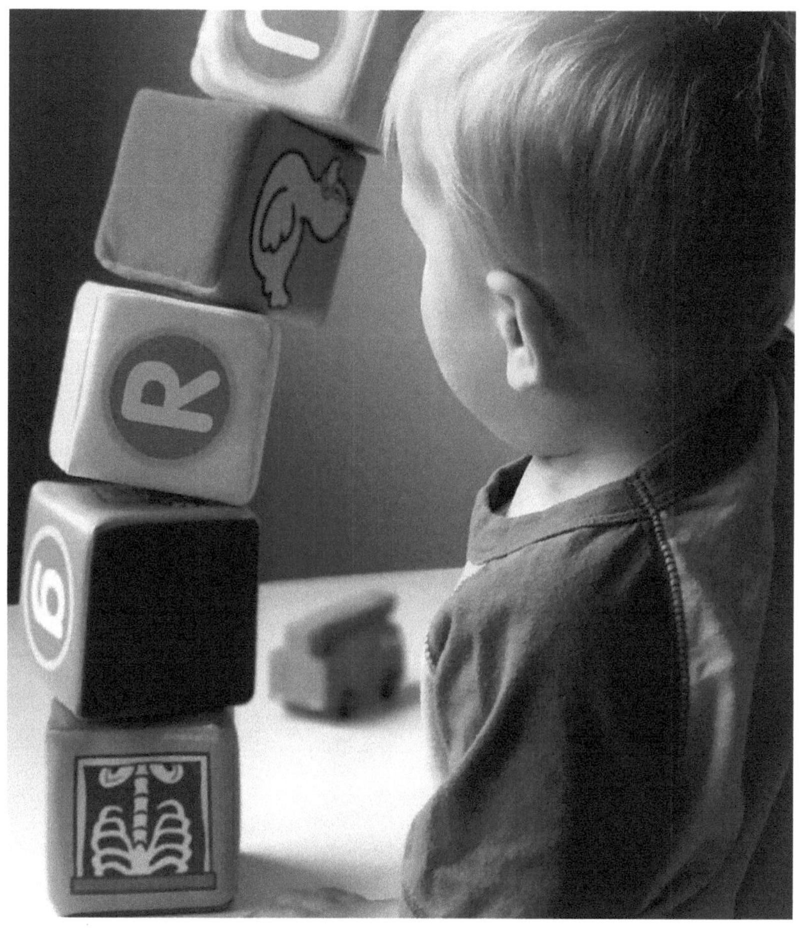

Autism Spectrum Disorder (ASD) has been widely discussed and investigated in the scientific literature due to the different levels of impairment in individuals, especially functional impairment. Multifactorial in nature, ASD is characterized by disorders of the neurological system, which lead to global developmental impairments, to a lesser or greater degree, according to diagnostic criteria.

According to data from the World Health Organization (WHO), one in every 160 children in the world is diagnosed with ASD. In the United States of America (USA), the figure is even higher. In 2022, according to the Centers for Disease Control and Prevention (CDC), it was estimated that every 30 children will be diagnosed with ASD, with males being four times more prevalent.

The word "autism" is of Greek origin and its meaning is related to the intrinsic behavior of individuals who are self-centered, which is why some symptoms are so recurrent and appear as early as the first two years of life. Despite this, the prevalence of diagnosis is between 5 and 8 years of age.

In order to make the diagnosis, it is necessary to consider the presence of behavioral manifestations and stereotypes presented by the child, especially in consultation with the pediatrician. The diagnosis is made with the help of screening tools, such as the Modified Checklist for Autism in Toddlers (M-CHAT), which was made compulsory by Law No. 13,438 of April 26, 2017, for children aged 16-30 months and is included in the 3rd edition of the child's booklet.

The M-CHAT questionnaire is intuitive and easy to use. It can be applied by pediatricians and other health professionals in a routine consultation. It consists of 23 questions, with yes/no answers and a final score: 0-2 points - low risk; 3-7 points – moderate risk; 8-20 points - high risk. Remember that as the M-CHAT is a screening tool, children should be referred to specialists, psychiatrists and/or child neurologists for diagnostic confirmation, as well as early intervention with a specialized multi-professional team for global development interventions in the necessary therapeutic areas.

The Brazilian Society of Pediatrics (SBP) and the American Academy of Pediatrics recommend that all children between the ages of 18 and 24 months be screened for ASD, even if they don't show any suggestive signs. The hope is that these children will be diagnosed earlier and benefit from therapeutic interventions, which are essential at this stage of neuroplasticity.

In ASD, difficulties in social interaction and communication, due to behavioral changes, the presence of hyperactivity, attention deficit, aggressiveness and sleep imbalances, can be associated with food and nutrition. In this context, nutritional disorders include food intolerances and allergies, restricted eating patterns, nutritional deficiencies, food selectivity, as well as gastrointestinal symptoms, which are quite common and can reach a prevalence of between 67 and 90% of children with ASD.

In the case of sleep disorders, also a recurring complaint from parents and caregivers, reduced melatonin production may be associated with autistic children, as shown in the recent study by Romeo et al. (2021), in which 46% of children with ASD had sleep disorders, compared to 15% of the control group, and this figure can reach 80% prevalence, depending on the variables analyzed. The reasons for these disorders point not only to a reduction in melatonin, but also in other neurotransmitters important for sleep, as well as behavioral and psychological factors.

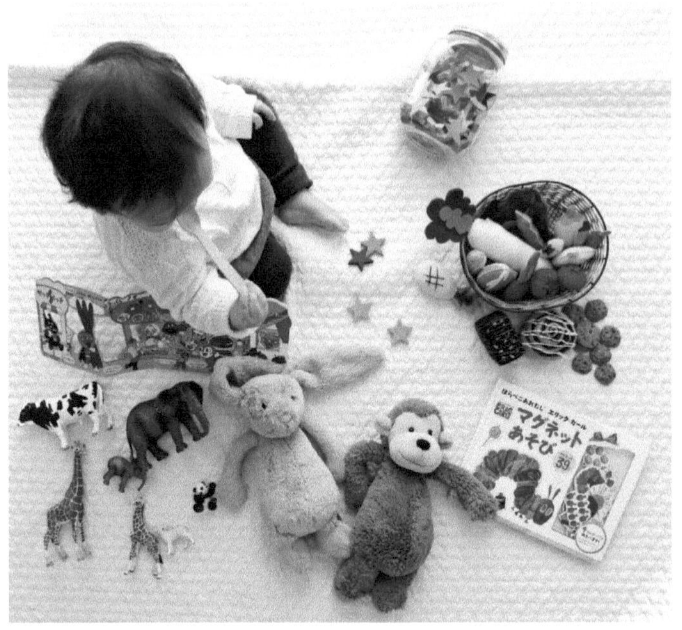

However, to date, there is no known cure for ASD, but there is strong evidence that diagnosis and early and preventive care can be a turning point in the treatment of these children. With the assistance of the nutritionist, together with the multidisciplinary team, nutritional and dietary strategies can have a positive and transformative influence on the quality of life of these children.

That's why, although a cure is unknown, it may be possible to change the prognosis of these children with ASD by easing their symptoms.

REFERENCES

AMERICAN PSYCHIATRIC ASSOCIATION [APA]. Manual
statistical diagnosis of mental disorders: DSM-V. 5 ed. Porto Alegre: Artmed; 2014.

GUEDES TAL. Free-to-use instruments for screening and classification of Autism Spectrum Disorders. SUS Open University. Federal University of Maranhão. São Luís: UNA-SUS; 2021.

KARHU E, et al. Nutritional interventions for autism spectrum disorder. Nutr Rev. 2020 Jul 1;78(7):515-531.

LI Q, LI Y, LIU B, et al. Prevalence of Autism Spectrum Disorder Among Children and Adolescents in the United States From 2019 to 2020, JAMA Pediatr. 2022;176(9):943-945.

MACIEL NGP. Addressing childhood autism in primary care: an integrative review. Revista Interdisciplinar em Saúde. 2020;7:466-481.

MAIA FA, ALMEIDA MT, ALVES MR, et al. Autism spectrum disorder and age of parents: a case-control study in Brazil. Cad. Saúde Pública. 2018; 34 (8).

MALHEIROS GC, PEREIRA MLC, et al. Benefits of early intervention in Autistic children. Revista Científica da FMC. 2017;12(1).

MODIFIED CHECKLIST FOR AUTISM IN TODDLERS (M-
CHAT) available at https://tn.gov/assets/entities/behavioral- health/attachments/ Pages_from_CY_BPGs_473-477.

MONTEIRO MA, SANTOS AA, GOMES LM, et al. Autism Spectrum Disorder: A Systematic

Review on Nutritional Interventions. Rev Paul Pediatr. 2020;38.

REDCAY E, COURCHESNE E. When Is the Brain Enlarged in Autism? A Meta-Analysis of All Brain Size Reports. Biol Psychiatry. 2005; 58:19.

REIS DL, NEDER PRB, MORAES MC, et al. Profile epidemiology of patients with Spectrum Disorder Autistic at the Specialized Rehabilitation Center. Res Med J. 2019;3(1):15.

SHARP WG, et al. Dietary Intake, Nutrient Status, and Growth Parameters in Children with Autism Spectrum Disorder and Severe Food Selectivity: an Electronic Medical Record Review. Journal of the Academy of Nutrition and Dietetics. 2018; 118(10):1943-1950.

SHARP WG, et al. Feeding problems and nutrient intake in children with autism spectrum disorders: a meta-analysis and comprehensive review of the literature. Journal of autism and developmental disorders. 2013; 43(9):2159-2173.

BRAZILIAN SOCIETY OF PEDIATRICS. Disorder of autism spectrum. Guidance Manual of the Scientific Department of Developmental and Behavioral Pediatrics. 2019;5.

CHAPTER 3

Nutritional Care for Children with ASD

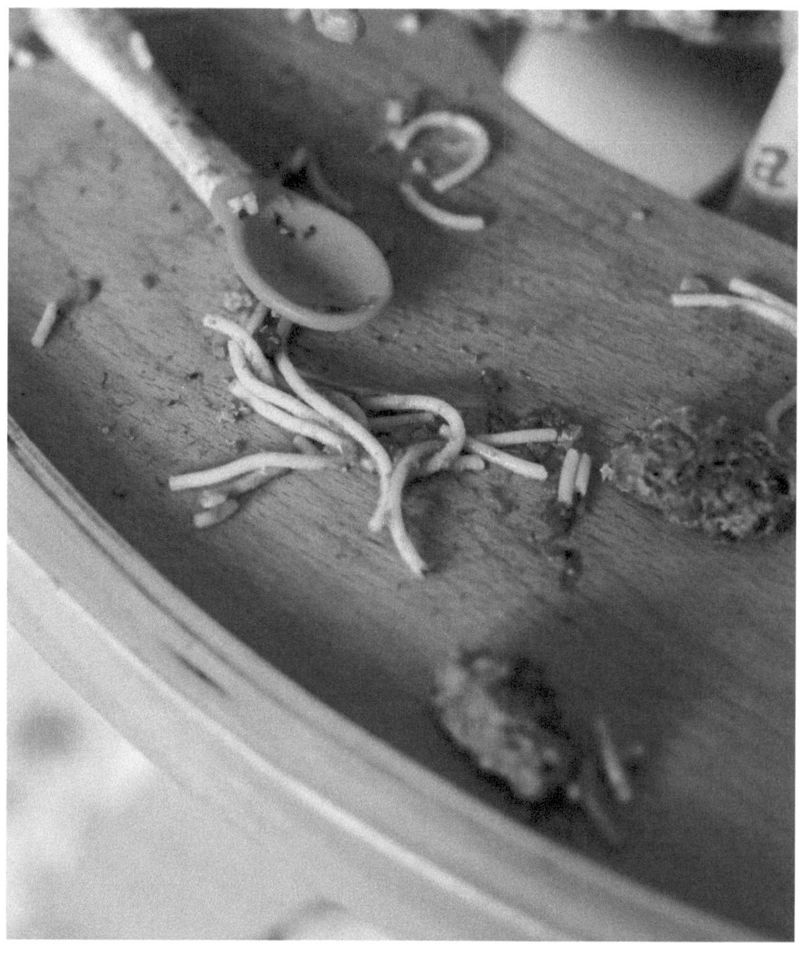

As yet, there are no specific nutritional guidelines or protocols for children with ASD, possibly due to the fact that this is a very heterogeneous group that responds in different ways to dietary treatment. In addition, the literature is quite divergent when it comes to measuring the effectiveness of each guideline and diet.

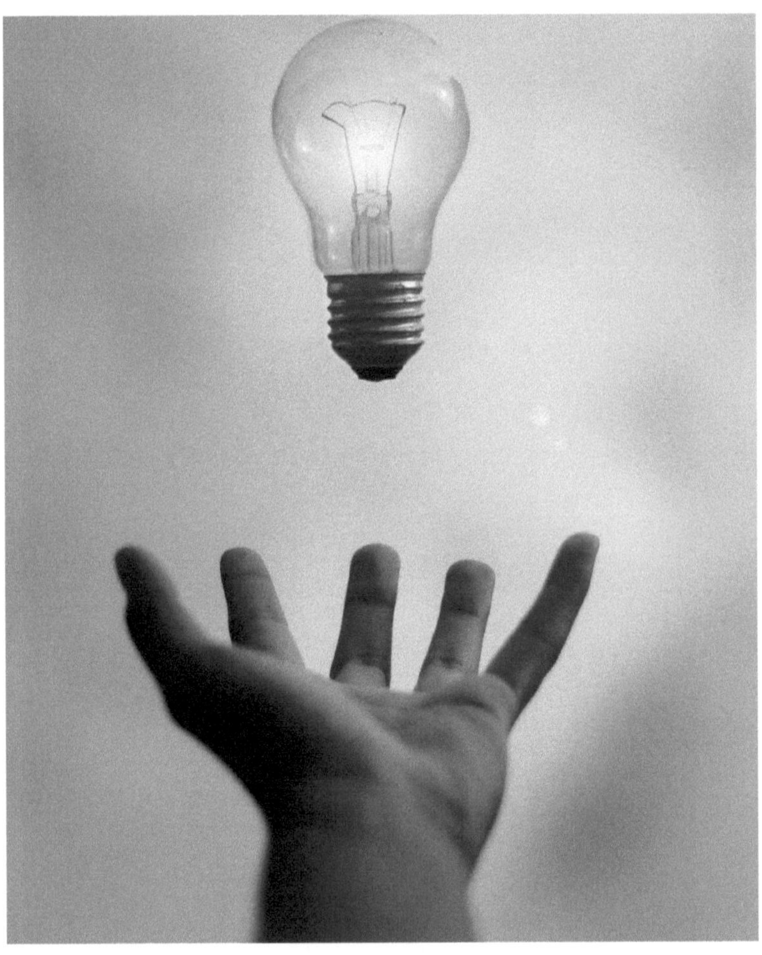

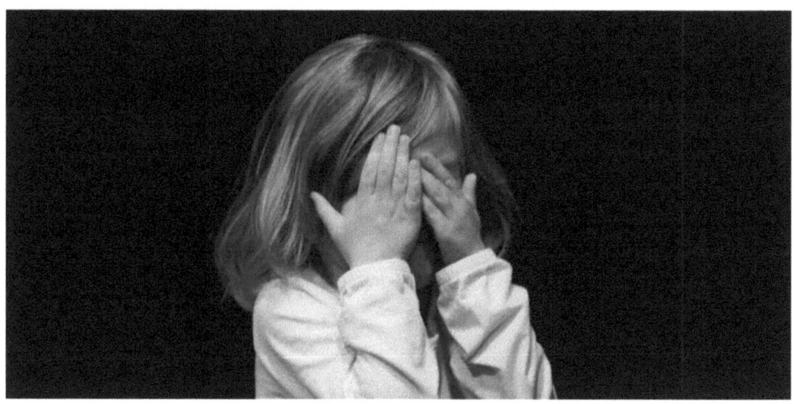

ASD symptoms related to food

a) Gastrointestinal tract

Gastrointestinal disorders are quite common in children with ASD and can account for up to 90% of family members' complaints. These disorders include epigastric pain, gastroesophageal reflux (GER), abdominal distension, flatulence, diarrhea or constipation. Symptoms such as these may be related to intestinal dysbiosis, given food allergies/intolerances, as well as increased intestinal permeability.

Dysbiosis occurs when there is an imbalance between the beneficial and pathogenic bacteria in the intestinal microbiome, leading to damage to the digestion and absorption of nutrients, especially high molecular weight proteins such as gluten and gliadin. With malabsorption, in addition to the classic symptoms, there can also be inflammation of the mucosa and the formation of neuropeptides that can cause neurological alterations in children with ASD.

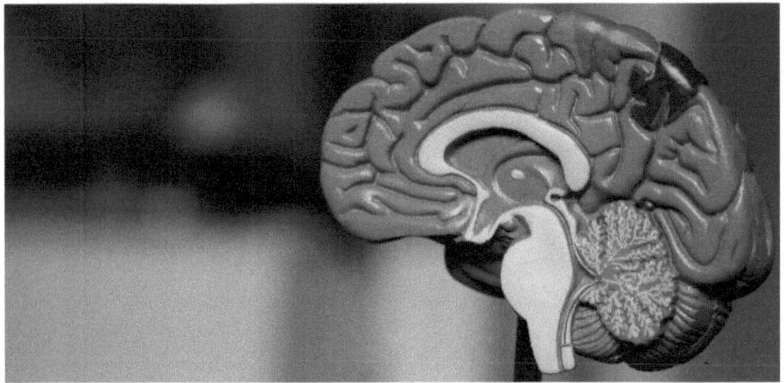

The hypothesis is that the abnormal metabolism of substances derived from incomplete digestion may generate bioactive peptides capable of crossing the blood-brain barrier and promoting neuroinflammation a n d the presence of the symptoms described.

Constipation is also common in children with ASD, as their consumption of dietary fiber is compromised. The reason for this manifestation may be due to dietary difficulties or selectivity, causing them to have a preference for foods with empty calories, food monotony and a diet rich in refined foods, which are very common in ultra-processed industrialized products.

Notwithstanding the unfavorable environmental context of these children, some studies have also shown that their antioxidant capacity seems to be compromised, with the involvement of genetic polymorphisms of antioxidant enzymes linked to serum SOD levels. Reduced levels of these enzymes can have a direct impact on the pathophysiology and progression of ASD symptoms.

b) Eating difficulties

They are characterized by any disorder that interferes with the child's feeding process, whether from organic causes, changes in sensory processing, motor abnormalities, gastrointestinal tract symptoms, the presence of food allergies/intolerances, abnormalities in the oral cavity or even behavioral issues, such as environments different from the usual ones, previous experiences in food introduction, bonding with the caregiver, as well as negative resources for feeding, such as forcing, manipulating or distracting. Family eating habits can also have an influence, such as the early introduction of ultra-processed foods containing high levels of sugar, sodium, saturated and trans fats, which stimulate the taste buds for such flavors, in the midst of the process of forming the baby's/child's eating habits.

In the case of food selectivity, restrictive eating patterns can be observed when the child chooses what to eat and separates food into categories, be they textures, colors, temperatures, smells, arrangement of food on the plate, use of specific utensils, choice of specific packaging for processed foods, among others.

Along with this behavior, there is a reduced appetite, refusal and lack of interest in new foods, as well as restriction by certain food groups, which makes the diet extremely unbalanced, increasing the chances of important nutritional imbalances and compromising the proper development of these children.

Nutritional imbalances generally include deficiencies in B vitamins, vitamin D and minerals such as iron, zinc and selenium, as well as deficiencies in essential fatty acids (omega 3), which can trigger an inflammatory cascade, with reduced immunity, the presence of repeat infections and exacerbation of behavioral and dietary symptoms.

However, even in the face of all these changes, the family context and environmental factors can play determining roles in these children's food choices, either by reinforcing food selectivity or by providing a more varied food environment in which nutritional strategies can be implemented in order to increase their repertoire.

Due to the complexity of the process of eating difficulties, any dietary intervention should be carried out naturally and gradually, in order to avoid negative feelings linked to mealtimes, such as agitation, aggression, spitting out food, throwing food on the floor, running away from food, self-injury and aggression towards caregivers. That moment, which should be pleasurable, ends up becoming violent and negatively impacting the introduction of healthy food, when this is the case. Furthermore, the treatment of selectivity is multifactorial, as already described, and multidisciplinary therapy is necessary to achieve beneficial results. It is necessary to work on cognitive, language, sensory and social skills.

That's why it's imperative to provide individualized care that is tailored to the needs of each child and family, because there is no "cake" recipe, but rather careful, integrated and daily work, so that progress can be made in a meaningful way. Building the best therapy is done by many hands.

Nutritional management in ASD

The nutritional management of children with ASD should initially be based on a healthy, balanced diet, made up of all the food groups, with low levels of sugar, sodium, trans and saturated fats, as recommended by the Food Guide for the Brazilian population.

However, we know that theory is far removed from practice when we meet children with atypical neurodevelopment. These demands require much more caution and individualization in dietary planning.

According to the literature, children with ASD tend to have altered nutritional status, usually with a prevalence of overweight and obesity, as well as macro and micronutrient deficiencies. This is due to dietary restrictions and the presence of food selectivity, as well as the rampant consumption of ultra-processed foods by this public. One of the reasons for this is that these children are more exposed to foods rich in sodium, fats and sugars and empty calories, as an attempt by family members and caregivers to get them to eat, regardless of nutritional quality. The practice of these deleterious habits not only stimulates the taste buds and neuronal receptors, but also interferes with the interest and introduction of healthy foods, exacerbating the disorders that are already in place.

It is necessary to carry out a complete and detailed nutritional anamnesis in order to investigate possible nutritional imbalances and make the necessary corrections, as well as to promote changes in the family's diet, especially when there are vices and bad habits that can contribute negatively and exacerbate the symptoms already presented. Generally speaking, the body needs to be balanced before any other type of intervention can begin.

Nutritional interventions have been a major focus of studies in recent years, especially with regard to their role in the symptoms presented by children with ASD. These include the ecological diet, consisting of antifungal foods with the inclusion of natural spices such as oregano, turmeric, thyme, coconut oil and seeds, as well as the removal of agrotoxins and pesticides; the FOODMAP-restricted diet, the purpose of which is to balance the intestinal microbiota, reducing flatulence by removing certain foods rich in monosaccharides (honey, fruit juice, corn syrup, etc.), disaccharides (milk and dairy products), oligosaccharides (flours) and polyols (xylitol, mannitol, sorbitol); the gluten- and casein-free diet (SGSC), which is one of the best known and most widely applied in clinical practice. This diet involves the removal of foods based on wheat, barley and rye flour and some types of oats (breads, cakes, pasta, cookies, cereals, cereal bars, among others) and dairy products (milk, cheese, cottage cheese, curd, sour cream), respectively.

What these diets have in common is the removal of certain foods and the substitution of others in order to soften/minimize symptoms. However, there is no robust scientific evidence to support this, and no food or food group should be removed without the assessment and recommendation of a qualified professional, as this could trigger other metabolic and nutritional imbalances. To this end, it is extremely important to check the real needs of each child, especially in cases of food sensitivities, allergies and/or intolerances, because food restrictions can also exacerbate the symptoms of food selectivity. Not all children will benefit from the alternative diets proposed.

With regard to sleep disorders in children with ASD, the presence of ultra-processed foods rich in sugar, caffeine, dyes, pesticides, preservatives, saturated fats, trans fats and sodium is under investigation, as the consumption of these foods is associated with increased production of free radicals and, consequently, oxidative stress, which could contribute significantly to neuronal inflammation and aggravation of autistic symptoms.

Clinical studies point to the presence of oxidative biomarkers, which have been shown to be deregulated in pediatric patients with autism. Evaluation of urinary and plasma levels of hexanoyl-lysine (HEL), the DNA methylation biomarker 8-hydroxy-2'-

deoxyguanosine (8-OHdG), superoxide dismutase (SOD) and total antioxidant capacity (TAOC) showed the presence of high levels of HEL and low levels of TAOC. It is also emphasized that diet can influence these results.

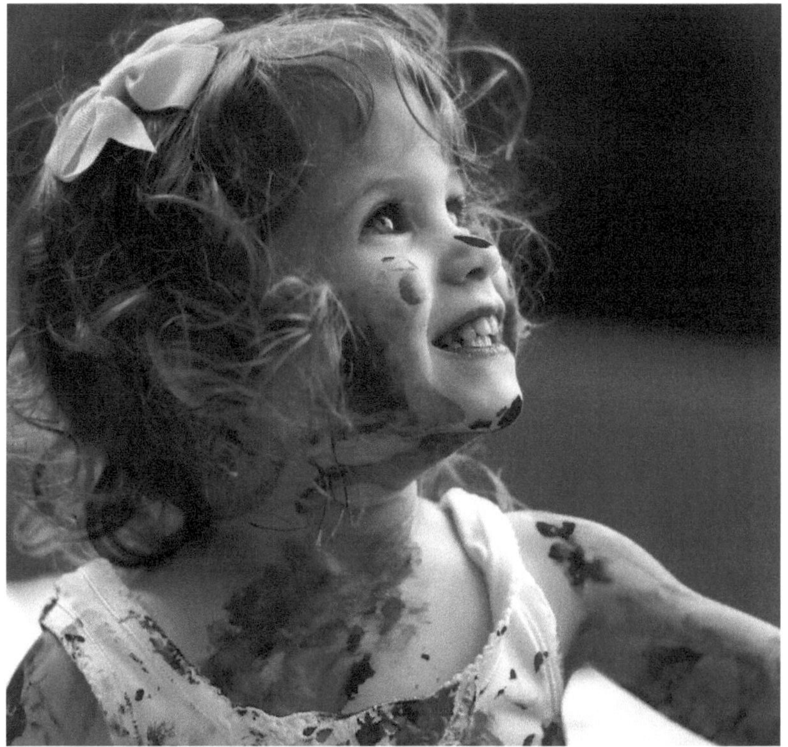

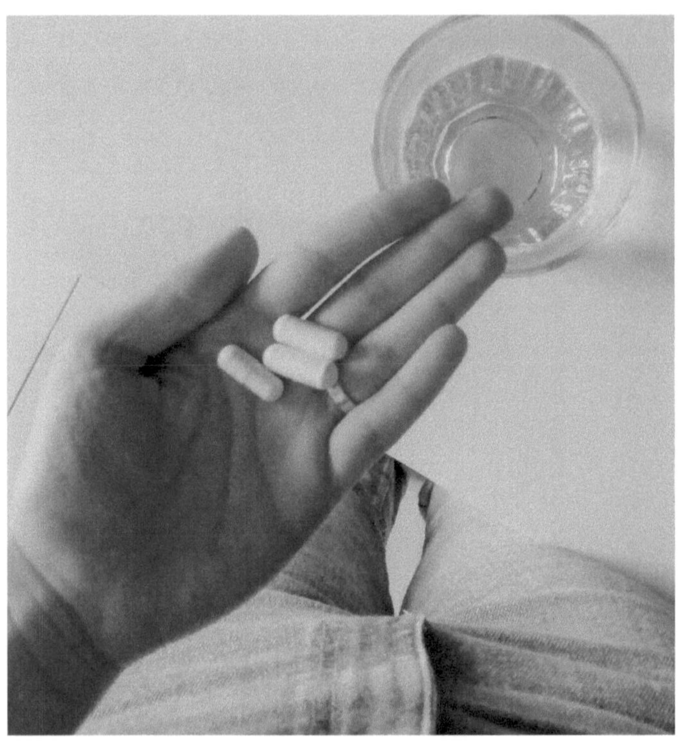

Supplementation... When to use it? Is it really necessary?

Nutritional supplementation can be an ally when used wisely and with caution, as it can correct nutritional imbalances in the body, as well as boosting compounds that would not be enough from food. When it comes to children with ASD, this modality becomes another positive point to be considered in the nutritional assessment process.

In order to do this, it is initially necessary to assess a few key factors before prescribing an exogenous nutrient: a) whether it is really necessary to correct needs that are not being met through dietary intake. The nutritional anamnesis will help in this investigation, based on a physical examination that allows us to check for signs of nutritional deficiency, request laboratory tests (B vitamins, vitamins A, C, D, zinc, selenium, iron, calcium, complete blood count, heavy metals and cortisol level, among others; b) adequacy of nutritional status, through weight and height according to age group, compared to the growth curves of the World Health Organization (WHO). Children with ASD have shown a prevalence of overweight (above the 85th percentile) and obesity (above the 97th percentile); c) whether the child has other diagnoses, such as allergy to cow's milk proteins (APLV), glucose-6-phosphate dehydrogenase (G6PD) deficiency, bronchitis, asthma and other respiratory disorders, conditions that can directly interfere with children's immunity, leaving them susceptible to pathogens entering the body, with greater exuberance of symptoms;

d) if gastrointestinal (GI) tract symptoms are present, such as flatulence, bloating, constipation or diarrhea.

In clinical practice, vitamins and minerals can be prescribed, which are usually not reached by food at first, especially if these children refuse to eat.

Hypercaloric and normoprotein supplements should be prescribed to children at risk of malnutrition, either because of associated diagnoses or because of the diet itself.

It is important to know the organization of the family routine and their eating habits. It is necessary to individualize each case, as well as understand the potential benefits of supplementation, as this modality must have specific and very clear purposes for its supporting role in the entire therapy of children with ASD, so that it can be properly measured and evaluated.

Nutraceuticals: what current studies say

- Probiotics and Prebiotics

Probiotics are a class of supplements made up of live, beneficial microorganisms that are essential for maintaining a healthy and balanced intestinal microbiota. As well as helping to absorb nutrients, they are also important for regulating the gut and immune system. Kefir and kombucha are common examples of probiotic supplements.

Prebiotics, on the other hand, are carbohydrates that cannot be digested by the GIT and which promote the growth of healthy microorganisms, leading to a balanced intestinal microbiota. Examples of prebiotics include whole grains, vegetables and fruit.

The use of probiotics and prebiotics by children with ASD is due to alterations in the GIT, known as intestinal dysbiosis. Studies have shown that neurotypical children can have an intestinal microbiota with a different composition of bacteria, which can usually be associated with this condition. In these children, the presence of clostridium and lactobacillus type bacteria is frequent, associated with restricted and repetitive behaviors.

In a study carried out by Wang et al. (2020), by analyzing the feces of autistic children, it was possible to observe that they had high levels of IgA, an important marker associated with immunity.

It is believed that probiotics, in addition to contributing to the restoration of immunity, can also reduce intestinal inflammation, marked by the presence of markers such as interleukin 1, 6, 13 and TNF-α, which are often found in patients with ASD.

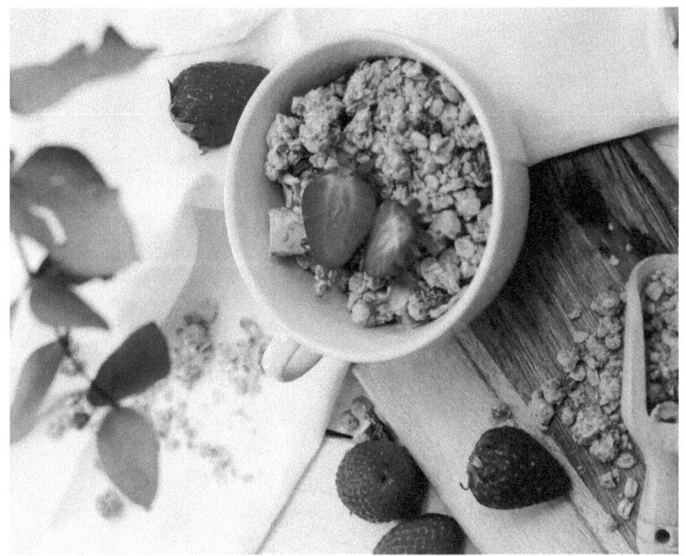

This reduces intestinal permeability and, consequently, the entry of undesirable microorganisms, and behavioral symptoms can also be minimized.

- VitaminD

Vitamin D3 (cholecalciferol) is produced primarily through exposure to sunlight (ultraviolet B rays - UVB). To a lesser extent, vitamin D3 can also be acquired through the diet by consuming foods of animal origin, such as fish, eggs, cod liver and dairy products. Vitamin D2 (calciferol) can be found in plant-based foods such as mushrooms and soya, as well as industrialized and fortified foods.

Although Brazil is a sunny country, it is quite common to find vitamin D deficiency, especially in the most vulnerable individuals, such as children and the elderly. In this sense, children with ASD are very vulnerable to vitamin D deficiency, which plays an important role in various regulatory processes in the body, including calcium metabolism, which is responsible for maintaining bone homeostasis and proper growth, as well as the immune and muscular systems, in addition to controlling chronic non-communicable diseases such as diabetes and systemic arterial hypertension (SAH).

Studies show that both children and adults with ASD have significantly lower levels of vitamin D when compared to neurotypical individuals. In addition, these lower levels of vitamin D have also been associated with exacerbation of symptoms such as hyperactivity and irritability. Furthermore, other studies show that vitamin D deficiency during pregnancy may be an increased risk for the birth of babies with ASD.

It is thought that adequate levels of vitamin D may have a protective effect on the regulation of inflammatory cytokines, raising the levels of important neurotransmitters such as serotonin and γ-aminobutyric acid (GABA).

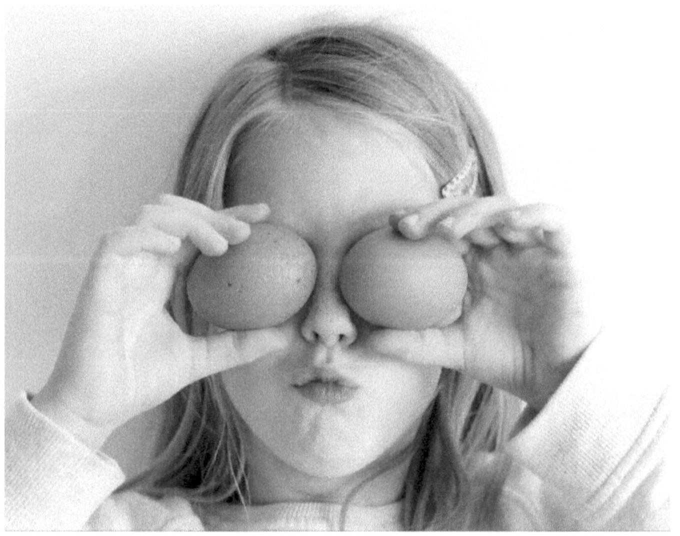

- Omega 3

Omega 3 is an essential polyunsaturated fatty acid, made up of alpha-linolenic acid (ALA), eicosapentaenoic acid (EPA) and docosahexaenoic acid (DHA). Its food sources are marine fish such as salmon, sardines and tuna, but it can also be found in linseed, chia seeds and extra virgin olive oil.

The numerous benefits of omega 3, especially DHA and EPA, have long been proven, as anti-inflammatory agents, promoters of cardiovascular health, reducers of joint pain, acting on cognitive functions and memory, among others.

Half of the human brain is made up of fat, so omega-3 fatty acids, particularly DHA, are essential for protecting neuronal membranes, promoting the healthy growth and development of neurons, as well as adequate synaptic connections. The literature highlights that omega-3 deficiency can directly influence the learning and cognition process.

Regarding the consumption of omega-3 by children with ASD, it is believed that there may be a positive influence due to the neuroprotective and antioxidant functions performed by omega-3. Furthermore, evidence also shows that children with ASD have lower levels of omega-3 compared to neurotypical children. This result may be related to the low dietary intake of omega-3, differences in fatty acid metabolism and incorporation into cell membranes in children with ASD.

Whatever the situation, these children can benefit from omega-3 supplementation, since this fatty acid is involved in concentration, agitation and learning. It is widely used in clinical practice and there have been reports of improvements in children's behavior, especially in relation to attention deficits.

- B-complex vitamins

Deficiencies of vitamins B6, B9 and B12 are not uncommon in children with ASD and may be due to low consumption, and occasionally, difficulties in metabolizing proteins of animal and vegetable origin, the main sources of which are meat, eggs, dairy products and legumes.

The B vitamins play an essential role in neurodevelopment, and severe deficiencies can compromise functions such as subsidizing the formation of neurons, biochemical reactions of methylation and sulphation, gross motor skills and language development. In particular, with vitamin B12 deficiency, there is an increase in serum and urine levels of methylmalonic and propionic acids, due to a metabolic shift, which is one of the causes of alterations in the central nervous system (CNS). Thus, symptoms of irritability, hyperactivity, attention deficit and sleep irregularities can result from these brain alterations.

Methylation reactions are essential for the activation of gene expression, acting both in the release of neurotransmitters and in the construction of flexible cell membranes for the entry of important nutrients from food and supplements, as well as for the excretion of toxic substances from the body. They also need B vitamins (B6, B9 and B12) for this process to take place.

Nutritional imbalances of this nature are of great relevance to public health and in this

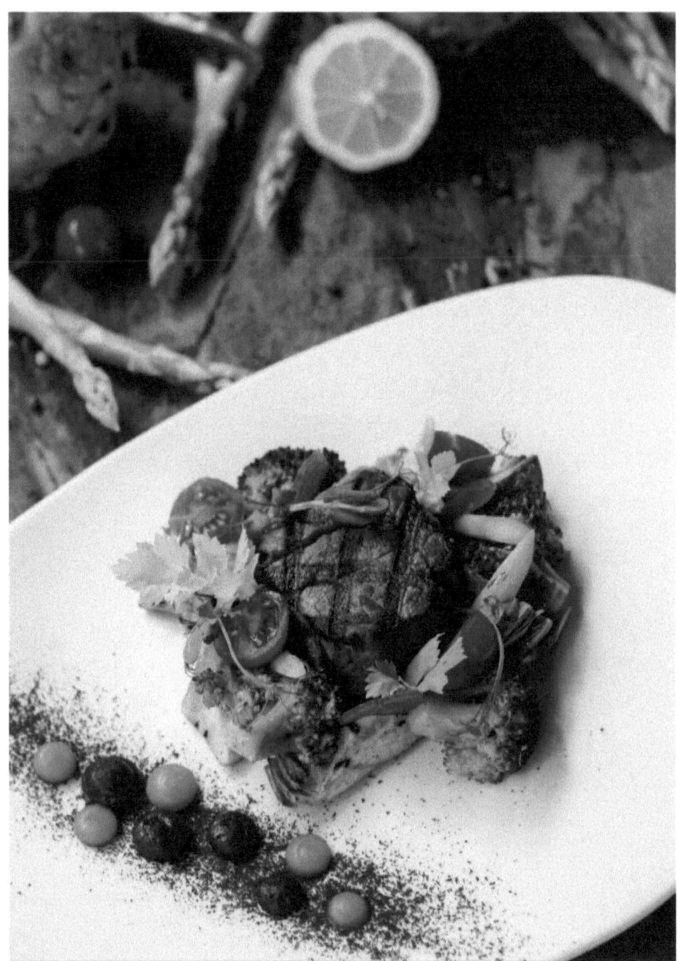

sense, the usual diet of autistic children is insufficient to meet all the demands of macro and micronutrients, which makes them eligible as a risk group for the development of nutritional deficiencies.

-The **association between heavy metals and ASD**

Heavy metals such as mercury, lead, cadmium and aluminum, found in food, contaminated water, pipes and paints, for example, are known for their toxicity in the body when individuals are exposed to or consume excessive sources.

Heavy metals are a group of chemical elements that are highly toxic, especially to the CNS. Children with ASD have difficulty combating the oxidative stress caused by these heavy metals, i.e. they are unable to detoxify efficiently due to low levels of glutathione (an important antioxidant for this process) and/or deregulated methylation and sulphation processes. In addition to this, it is possible that the gene expression of children with ASD influences the behavior of heavy metals in their bodies.

Supplementation with trace elements such as selenium can lead to greater antioxidant capacity, as well as reducing the inflammatory response of epithelial cells by regulating inflammatory cytokines such as TNF-α and IL-6. With regard to children with ASD, the neuroinflammation in the hippocampus and frontal lobes stands out, as they have reduced levels of trace elements such as zinc, selenium, magnesium and calcium in their bodies, when analyzed in hair, nail and blood samples.

REFERENCES

AL-KINDI NM, AL-FARSI Y, AL-BULUSHI B, t al. Food
Selection and Preferences of Omani Autistic Children. NEUROBIOL. 2020; 24: 515-533.

ALMEIDA AKA, FONSECA PCA, et al. Consumption of ultra-processed foods and nutritional status of children with autism spectrum disorder. Revista Brasileira em Promoção da Saúde. 2018; São Luís, Maranhão, Brazil.

ÂNGELO KHA, FILHO PFS, et al. Nutritional supplementation as a therapeutic approach in autism spectrum disorder: A literature review. Research, Society and Development. 2021; 10 (9).

AUDISIO A, LAGUZZI J, et al. Improvement of autism symptoms and nutritional dietary assessment after the implementation of a gluten- and casein-free diet in a group of children with autism attending a foundation. Nutr. clin. diet. hosp. 2013; 33(3):39-47.

BABINSKA K, et al. Gastrointestinal Symptoms and Feeding Problems and Their Associations with Dietary Interventions, Food Supplement Use, and Behavioral Characteristics in a Sample of Children and Adolescents with Autism Spectrum Disorders. Int J Environ Res Public Health. 2020; 17(17).

BALBONI MCH, GOWDAK MMG, et al. Impact of Omega-3 Fatty Acids Supplementation on Autism Spectrum Disorders: Systematic Review Based on Randomized Controlled Clinical Trials. Rev Soc Cardiol Estado de São Paulo. 2019;29(2):203- 10.

BOTTAN GP, DUARTE CN, SANTANA JRS. Analyzing the

feeding autistic people through a literature review. Braz. J. of Develop. 2020; 12(6): 100448-100470.

BRANDÃO MF, COSTA AN, et al. Socioeconomic, demographic and nutritional characteristics of children with autism spectrum disorder. Demetra, Alimentação Nutrição&Saúde. 2023.

BRANDÃO TLS et al. Prebiotic and probiotic supplementation in autistic children: integrative review. Research, Society and Development. 2022; 11 (1).

CARVALHO MF, SANTANA MZ. Food and Nutrition Education for children with Autism Spectrum Disorder: a proposal for practical activities at school, in the clinic and at home. Recife. Pró-Reitoria de Extensão e Cultura da UFPE; Ed. UFPE. 2022.

CUPERTINO MC, RESENDE MB, VELOSO IF, et al.

Autism spectrum disorder: a systematic review on nutritional aspects and the gut-brain axis. ABCS Health Sci. 2019; 44(2):120-130.

DARGENIO VN, DARGENIO C, CASTELLANETA S, et al.

Intestinal Barrier Dysfunction and Microbiota-Gut-Brain Axis: Possible Implications in the Pathogenesis and Treatment of Autism Spectrum Disorder. Nutrients. 2023 Apr; 15(7): 1620.

DIERINGS L, DESIDÉRIO NC, MATTIELLO S. Prevalence

of vitamin B12 deficiency in patients of a clinical analysis laboratory in Francisco Beltrão, PR. Acta Elit Salutis. 2020; 2(1).

FENG J, SHAN L, et al. The association of vitamin A, zinc and Copper levels with clinical symptoms in children with autism spectrum disorders in Jilin Province, China. BMC Pediatrics. 2023; 23:173.

FIGUEROLA PE, CANALS J, FERNÁNDEZ JC. Differences in food consumption and nutritional intake between children with autism spectrum disorders and typically developing children: A meta-analysis. Autism. 2019; 23(5): 1079-1095.

GHALICHI F, GHAEMMAGHAMI F, MALEK A, OSTADRAHIMI A. Effect of gluten free diet on gastrointestinal and behavioral indices for children with autism spectrum disorders: a randomized clinical trial. World J Pediatr. 2016 Nov;12(4):436-442.

İLERI SE, ÇELIKKOL CS, et al. Serum B12, homocysteine, and anti-parietal cell antibody levels in children with autism. International Journal of Psychiatry in Clinical Practice. 2021.

INFANTE M, SEARS B, et al. Omega-3 PUFAs and vitamin D co-supplementation as a safe-effective therapeutic approach for core symptoms of autism spectrum disorder: case report and literature review. Nutritional Neuroscience.2018.

KANG DW et al. Microbiota transfer therapy alters the gut ecosystem and improves gastrointestinal and autism symptoms: an open study. Microbiome. 2017; 5 (1): 1-16.

LASHERAS I, LÓPES MR, SANTABÁRBARA J. Prevalence of gastrointestinal symptoms in autism spectrum disorder: A meta-analysis. Anales de Pediatría. 2023; 99 (2): 102-110.

LEADER G, ABBERTON C, CUNNINGHAM S, et al.
Gastrointestinal Symptoms in Autism Spectrum Disorder: A Systematic Review. Nutrients 2022;14(7):1471.

MARTINS H, MOLINA B, et al. Intestinal microbiota and its relationship with autism: an integrative review. Concilium. 2022; 22 (6): 699-710.

MONTEIRO MA, SANTOS AA, GOMES LM, et al. Autism Spectrum Disorder: A Systematic Review on Nutritional Interventions. Rev Paul Pediatr. 2020;38.

MOREIRA P, SANTOS S, et al. Food Patterns According to Sociodemographics, Physical Activity, Sleeping and Obesity in Portuguese Children. Int. J. Environ. Res. Public Health. 2010; 7: 1121-1138.

MUNOZ RG. Clinical features suggestive of autistic spectrum disorder as a manifestation of non-celiac gluten sensitivity. Servicio de Neonatología, Hospital Universitario Materno-Infantil de Las Palmas de Gran Canaria, Las Palmas de Gran Canaria. Spain. 2014.

NEME G, RODRIGUES CS, et al. Autism Spectrum Disorder and Heavy Metals: A Systematic Review. Revista UNILUS Ensino e Pesquisa. 2020; 17(46): 120.

PAIVA GSJ, et al. Nutritional education and autism: which way forward? Raízes e Rumos. 2020; 8(2): 98 - 114.

PALLEJA`AV, TORRELL H, et al. Genetic and clinical evidence of mitochondrial dysfunction in autism spectrum disorder and intellectual disability. Human Molecular Genetics.

2018; 27 (5): 891-900.

PENAFORTE NF, VASCONCELOS CAC, BARBOSA AK.
Possible relationship between dietary changes in micronutrients and behavioral symptoms in autism spectrum disorder. Memorial Journal of Medicine. 2019; 1(2):37-45.

RASHIDY O, BAZ F, et al. Ketogenic diet versus gluten free casein free diet in autistic children: a case-control study. Metab BrainDis. 2017.

REDCAY E, COURCHESNE E. When Is the Brain Enlarged in Autism? A Meta- Analysis of All Brain Size Reports. Biol Psychiatry. 2005; 58:1-9.

RESTREPO B, ANGKUSTSIRI K, TAYLOR SL, et al.
Developmental-behavioral profiles in children with autism spectrum disorder and co-occurring gastrointestinal symptoms. Autism Res. 2020;13(10):1778-1789.

ROCHA GS, LIMA ND, LIMA MS, et al. Alternative and complementary therapies in the treatment of gastrointestinal symptoms in children with Autism Spectrum Disorder. Revista Eletrônica Acervo Saúde. 2020; 52:1-10.

RODRIGUES CPS, SILVA JPA, ÁLVARES IQ. Autism is correlated with sensory-oral changes and eating behavior. Braz. J. of Develop. 2020; 6(9): 67155-67170.

SABINO SMV, BELÉM MO. The relationship between autism spectrum disorder and intestinal dysbiosis: an integrative review. J. Health Biol Sci. 2022;10(1):1-9.

SANTOS JS, SILVA RB, SILVA DCB. Food consumption, according to degree of processing, of children and adolescents with autism spectrum disorder. Braz. J. of DeveloP. 2020; 6(10): 83322-83334.

SATHE N, ANDREWS JC, MCPHEETERS ML, et al.
Nutritional and Dietary Interventions for Autism Spectrum
Disorder: A Systematic Review.Pediatrics. 2017;139(6).

SMAGA I, NIEDZIELSKA E, GAWLIK M, et al. Oxidative
stress as an etiological factor and a potential treatment target of psychiatric disorders. Part 2: Depression, anxiety, schizophrenia and autism. Pharmacological Reports. 2015; 67: 569-580.
BRAZILIAN SOCIETY OF PEDIATRICS. Manual of
guidelines for feeding infants, preschoolers, schoolchildren, adolescents and children at school. Brazilian Society of Pediatrics. Department of Nutrology. 2012;1(3).

SWEETMAN DU, O'DONNELL SM, et al. Zinc and vitamin A deficiency in a cohort of children with autism spectrum disorder. Child Care Health Dev. 2019;45(3):380-6.

WANG Y, et al. Probiotics and fructo-oligosaccharide intervention modulate the microbiota-gut brain axis to improve autism spectrum reducing also the hyper-serotonergic state and the dopamine metabolism disorder. Pharmacological research. 2020
.

WU H, ZHAO G, et al. Supplementation with selenium attenuates autism-like behaviors and improves oxidative stress, inflammation and related gene expression in an autism disease model. The Journal of Nutritional Biochemistry. 2022; 107: 109034.

YUIA K, TANUMA N, YAMADA H, et al. Reduced

endogenous urinary total antioxidant power and its relation of plasma antioxidant activity of

superoxide dismutase in individuals with autism spectrum disorder. Int. J.Devl

Neuroscience. 2016.

CHAPTER 4:

Food and Nutrition Education for Children with ASD

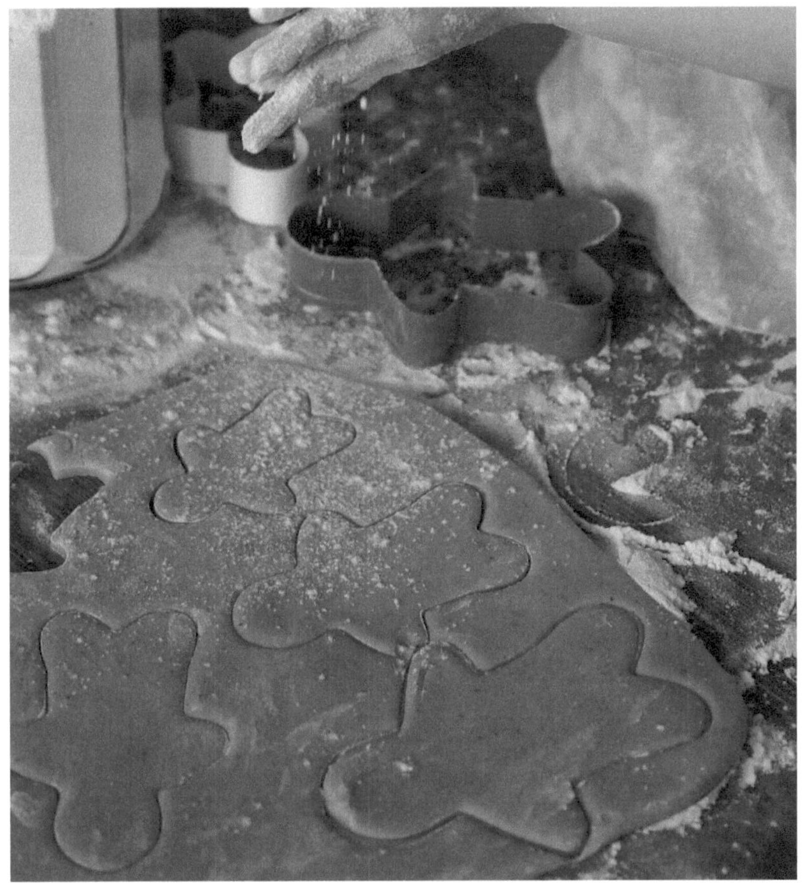

Food and Nutrition Education (FNE) is a strategy that considers the cultural, social and economic influence on people's food choices, encouraging the appreciation of food as an essential element for life, with the aim of promoting the construction of adequate and healthy knowledge and habits about food and nutrition, which provide health and quality of life.

EAN stands out in the context of the National Food and Nutrition Policy (PNAN), as a fundamental part of achieving users' protagonism and emancipation over their health, as well as being an efficient, safe, easy-to-use approach that makes it possible to explore a

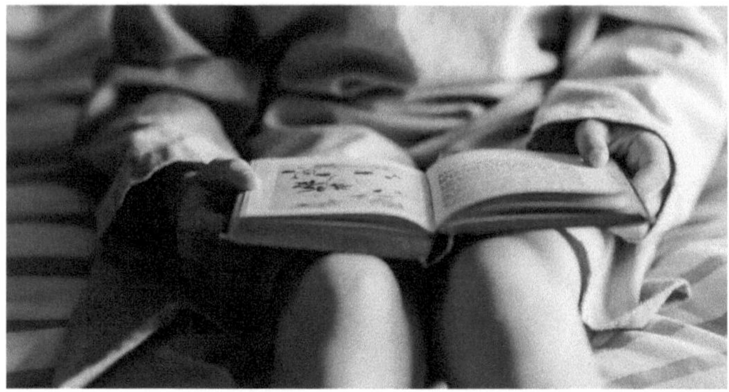

diversity of resources. It is presented as a nutritional intervention capable of overcoming the challenges related to food and nutrition in ASD, making it necessary to involve family members and people close to them in EAN educational practices and, consequently, dietary changes, given their influence on children's eating behavior.

It has long been recognized how beneficial early intervention in ASD can be for its clinical outcome, which makes nutritional education actions as part of therapeutic treatment paramount, aiming not only for the best prognosis for these children, but also as a way of exponentially expanding knowledge among health professionals, education, parents and the community, under a more integrated, networked framework, in which everyone really does have access to the same treatment, with all the benefits they are entitled to.

In order to include educational nutritional activities, family participation is essential, since children learn by example and habits at home from a very young age.

In this way, these experiences should denote pleasure, opportunities, meaning and affection in how these foods are presented from the moment they are introduced, determining the child's behavior towards food.

The nutritionist, a key educator and specialist in this process, should be involved in helping these families with preventive strategies, to avoid eating behaviors that could characterize an erroneous diet, rich in sodium, sugars and saturated fats, often introduced hastily as a last resort to get the child to eat.

The success of EAN depends on understanding the process, which requires patience, understanding and several attempts. It cannot be neglected by any party. For a satisfactory result to occur, family, school and therapists must be in harmony.

In this sense, continuing and ongoing education activities are needed for parents and caregivers, such as nannies, grandparents, teachers, involving topics pertinent to the incorporation of healthy eating habits, including knowledge about minimally processed, processed and ultra-processed foods; reading food labels; making use of all parts of food; culinary workshops with food chaining; benefits and nutrients present in food, as well as free topics, all according to the doubts and suggestions of family members and caregivers, among others.

After this stage, the children's presence at the nutritional education activities will be the thermometer for choosing which path to follow and which activities to choose, given that they are a heterogeneous group and will not necessarily respond in the same way to the proposed activities. However, some strategies are extremely important for the majority of cases: concrete activities, using familiar tools that denote attachment and/or affinity on the part of the child; activities and foods presented in different ways, several times, not consecutively; active participation in the whole process, from choosing the food to work on to preparing a meal; activities that use everyday life to resemble the routine already established and accepted by the child at home; use of colors, textures; utensils, such as cutlery, plates and glasses; and toys of preference. The activities should be playful and adapted to arouse the child's interest.

In general, the nutritionist, as an intermediary in this process, should work together with the interdisciplinary team, family members and caregivers, and the child themselves, to promote a welcoming, pleasant environment that values healthy habits and encourages changes at home. It is essential that children feel comfortable at mealtimes, that they are understood and respected, so that they can gradually expand their eating repertoire.

REFERENCES

CARVALHO MF, SANTANA MZ. Food and Nutrition Education for children with Autism Spectrum Disorder: a proposal for practical activities at school, in the clinic and at home. Recife. Pro-Rectory of Extension and Culture of UFPE; Ed. UFPE. 2022.

FRANÇA CJ, SANTOS VCH. Food and nutrition education strategies in Primary Health Care: a literature review. Saúde em Debate. 2017;114(41).

MINISTRY OF HEALTH. National Food and Nutrition Policy. Department of Primary Care. 1ed. Brasília: Ministry of Health, 2013.

MONTEIRO MA, SANTOS AA, GOMES LM, et al. Autism Spectrum Disorder: A Systematic Review on Nutritional Interventions. Rev Paul Pediatr. 2020;38.

MONTEIRO MA, SANTOS AA, GOMES LM, et al. Autism Spectrum Disorder: A Systematic Review on Nutritional Interventions. Rev Paul Pediatr. 2020;38.

PAIVA GSJ, et al. Nutritional education and autism: which way forward? Raízes e Rumos. 2020; 8(2): 98 - 114.

PRADO BG, FORTES ENS, LOPES MAL. Food and nutrition education actions for schoolchildren: an experience report. Demetra. 2016;11(2):369-382.

BRAZILIAN SOCIETY OF PEDIATRICS. Guidance manual for feeding infants, preschoolers, schoolchildren, adolescents and children at school. Brazilian Society of Pediatrics. Department of Nutrology. 2012;1(3).

SOUZA LMS, SANTOS SMC. National Food and Nutrition Policy: evaluation of the implementation of programs in municipalities in Bahia. Demetra: alimentação, nutrição &saúde. 2017; 12(1); 137-155.

This *e-book* highlights the strengths and reflections of diet therapy applied to children with ASD.

The nutritionist, together with the interdisciplinary team, is key to building and transforming eating habits, especially when nutritional disorders are present.

However, the multifactorial complexity of ASD requires constant vigilance and monitoring of these children, so that they have the right to adequate food, consisting of all the essential nutrients for their healthy development, guaranteeing their right to food and nutritional security.

Finally, we hope to contribute to increasing and reinforcing the knowledge and practices of health professionals who assist children with ASD.

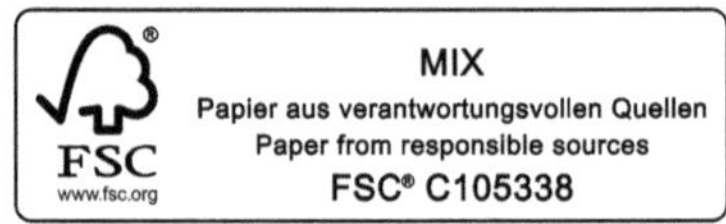

Printed by Books on Demand GmbH, Norderstedt / Germany